Acknowledgements

The author wishes to thank Dr. Raúl Sánchez Sánchez and Dr. Ernesto Gómez Fidalgo, researchers at the Department of Animal Reproduction of the National Institute for Agricultural and Food Research and Technology (INIA) (Madrid, Spain), for their authorisation to visit the facilities in their centre, and Dr. Juan Carlos Fontanillas Pérez, Professor at the Department of Animal Physiology of the School of Veterinary Medicine of the Complutense University of Madrid, for his help in obtaining the photographic material for this handbook.

Author

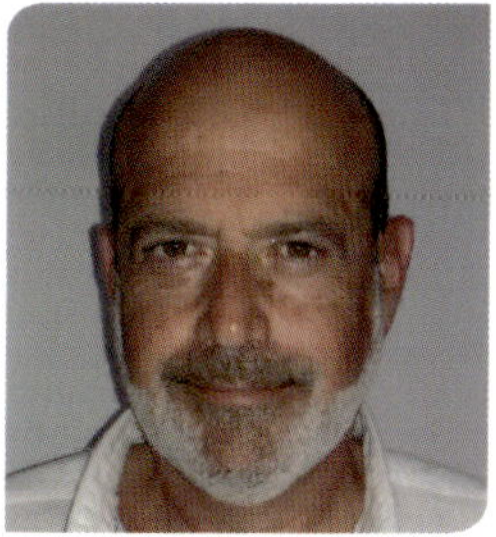

Carlos García Artiga

Ldo. Vet, PhD

Associate Professor at the Zoology teaching unit of the Department of Physiology (Animal Physiology), Faculty of Veterinary Medicine, Complutense University of Madrid (UCM), Spain.

Coordinators

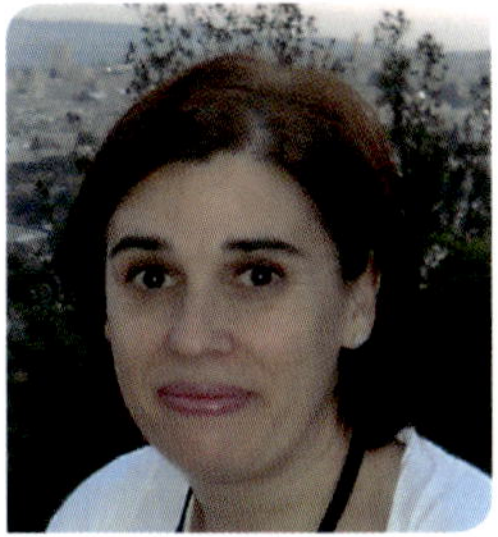

Rosa María García García

Lda. Vet, PhD

Associate Professor at the Department of Physiology (Animal Physiology) of the Faculty of Veterinary Medicine, UCM, Spain.

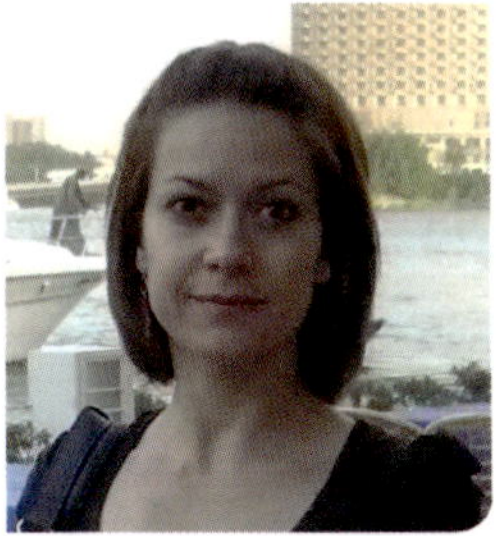

María Arias Álvarez

Lda. Vet, PhD

Associate Professor at the Department of Animal Production at the Faculty of Veterinary Medicine of the UCM, Spain.

TABLE OF CONTENTS

Semen collection and processing

1 Introduction

Artificial insemination (AI) has long been a routine practice in pig breeding. It allows the use of genetically selected boars and improves rates of fertility and prolificacy on breeding farms. The boar has a major impact on reproductive efficiency, given that the semen of a single individual can be used to inseminate between 750 and 1,000 sows per year using traditional AI approaches, and sperm quality is directly correlated with fertility.

Thanks to advances in the techniques used to administered sperm doses, the sperm concentration in insemination doses has been reduced from $3{,}000 \times 10^6$ to $1{,}500 \times 10^6$. The control and monitoring of the quality of ejaculates for artificial insemination is thus even more important now than ever before.

Optimal management of boars is essential to ensure the reproductive efficiency of the farm.

The use of high-quality ejaculate in AI decreases the number of boars that are maintained on the farm and allows a better optimisation of the fertility rate. Currently, 90 % of AI in swine production is carried out using semen that is diluted, refrigerated and stored at 15–17 °C for 1 to 6 days. Using a practical approach, this book reviews the different phases and key elements in AI: the area used to train boars and collect semen, the collection methods, the assessment of sperm quality and quantity, and semen processing and storage.

Anatomy

The reproductive tract of the male pig consists of several structures: the testes, epididymis, accessory sex glands, duct system, and penis (Fig. 1).

The main functions of the testes are to produce spermatozoa and secrete hormones, while the epididymis is responsible for the transport, maturation and storage of semen. The prostate, seminal vesicles, and bulbourethral glands (Cowper's glands) comprise the accessory sex glands, which are involved in the production of seminal plasma. Therefore, the ejaculate is composed mainly of sperm and seminal plasma.

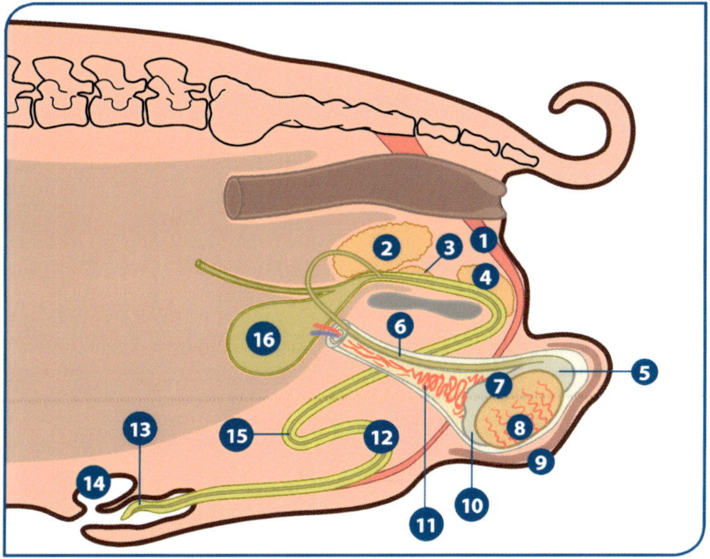

Figure 1. Reproductive tract of the male pig.

1. Retractor penis muscle
2. Vesicular glands
3. Prostate gland
4. Bulbourethral glands
5. Tail of epididymis
6. Vas deferens
7. Body of epididymis
8. Testis
9. Scrotum
10. Head of epididymis
11. Spermatic cord
12. Sigmoid flexure of penis
13. Glans penis
14. Preputial diverticulum
15. Penile urethra
16. Bladder

Hypothalamic-pituitary-gonadal axis

Reproductive activity is controlled by the endocrine and nervous systems. The testes receive information via the hypothalamic-pituitary-gonadal axis (Fig. 2). The hypothalamus produces GnRH, which induces the release of LH and FSH from the adenohypophysis. FSH acts directly on germ cells and on the Sertoli cells of seminiferous tubules in the testes, stimulating spermatogenesis. LH stimulates the production of androgens in the Leydig cells in the testes. Testosterone, the main androgen, stimulates and regulates sperm production and male sexual behaviour. Inhibin (secreted by the Sertoli cells) has a negative feedback effect on FSH secretion; testosterone inhibits the release of GnRH, which in turn reduces LH secretion.

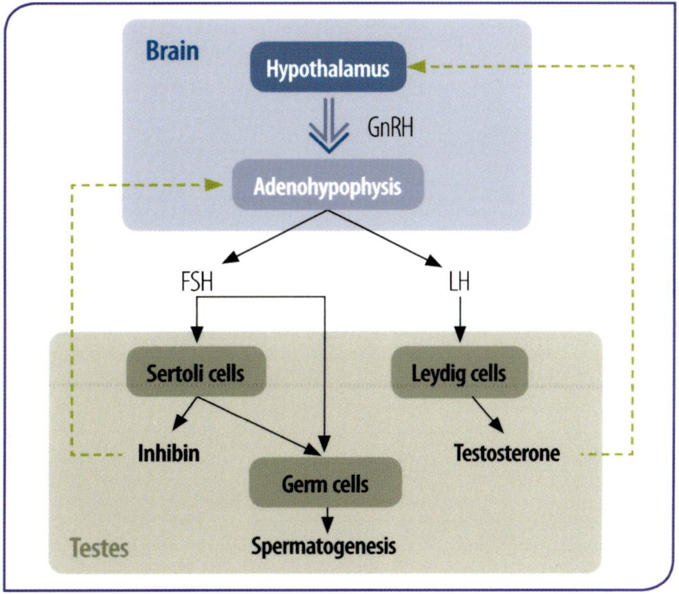

Figure 2. Hypothalamic-pituitary axis. The hypothalamus produces GnRH, which stimulates the release of FSH and LH from the adenohypophysis to regulate the production of testosterone (T), spermatogenesis, and male sexual behaviour. Dashed lines indicate inhibition while solid lines indicate stimulation.

Spermatogenesis

Spermatogenesis is an extremely complex process, which involves the constant production of spermatozoa in the seminiferous tubules of the testes. In the adult boar, the testicular parenchyma consists of two compartments: tubular and intertubular compartments (Figs. 3 and 4).

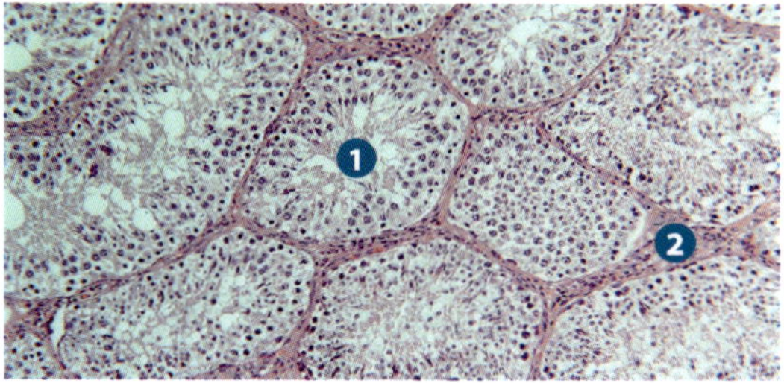

Figure 3. Histological section of the testes of an adult boar. Tubular compartment (seminiferous tubules) containing Sertoli cells and germ cells (1), and intertubular compartment (interstitial tissue) (2) containing Leydig cells and blood vessels (10×).

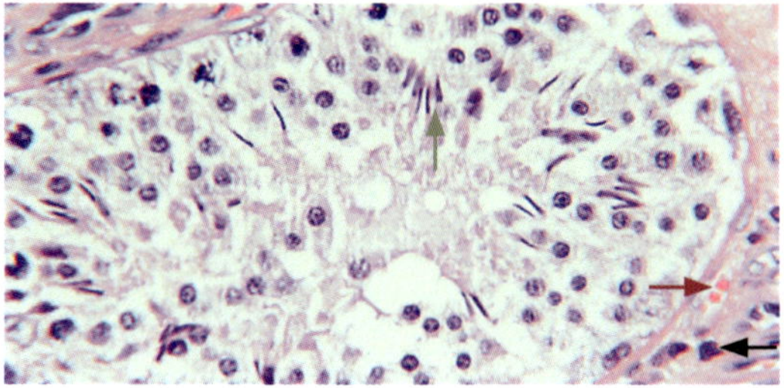

Figure 4. Detail of a seminiferous tubule containing Sertoli cells and germ cells in differents stages, elongated spermatids (green arrow) and intertubular compartment containing Leydig cells (black arrow) and blood vessels (red arrow) (40×).

- The tubular compartment, composed of seminiferous epithelium and containing Sertoli cells and germ cells in different stages of development.
- The intertubular compartment, which contains a large number of Leydig cells and blood vessels.

In boars, the process of spermatogenesis takes about 35 to 40 days and transit of spermatozoa through the epididymis approximately 9 to 14 days (6–8 days in the head and body of the epididymis and storage in the tail for approximately 8 days; Fig. 5).

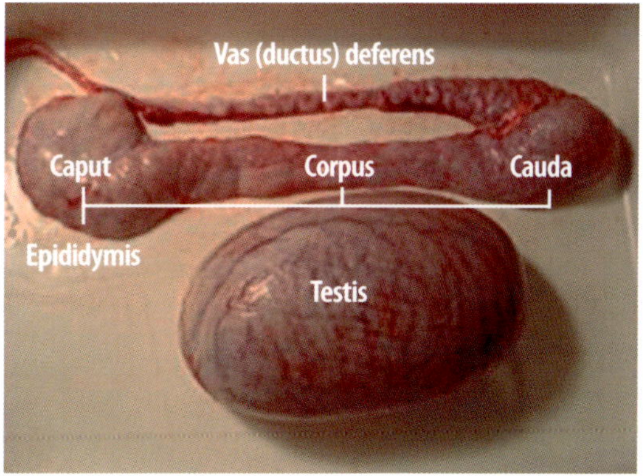

Figure 5. Testes and epididymis of an adult boar. The spermatozoa travel from the head (caput) to the tail (cauda) of the epididymis in a process that takes between 9 and 14 days. About 75 % of the spermatozoa contained in the epididymis is found in the tail.

Reproductive development

Spermatogenesis and testicular development begin during the early embryonic life. Reproductive behaviour starts during the first month of life, and puberty occurs at 5 to 6 months of age, accompanied by an increase in semen production (Table 1). However, males cannot be used for reproductive purposes until a few months later, as during puberty they produce a low volume of ejaculate, containing a low sperm count and primarily immature spermatozoa.

Table 1. Reproductive maturation in the boar (Knox, 2003).

Maturation process	Age
Division and differentiation of germ cells	Foetus (20–40 days)
Descent of testes from the abdomen into the scrotum	Foetus (60 days)
Mounting behaviour	1–2 months
Second division of germ cells and increase in the relative size of the testes	3 months
Sperm in the seminiferous tubules. Erections may be observed	4 months
Onset of puberty and presence of sperm in ejaculate	5 months
Increase in the testicular size, sperm concentration, and the volume of ejaculate	6–18 months

Introduction

The semen collection and boar training room should be designed in accordance with animal welfare regulations. In Europe, legislation stipulates that boars should be provided with an individual enclosure in which they can turn around and hear, smell, and see other boars (Fig. 1). If the same area is used for service, the space should be at least 10 m^2 and free of obstacles.

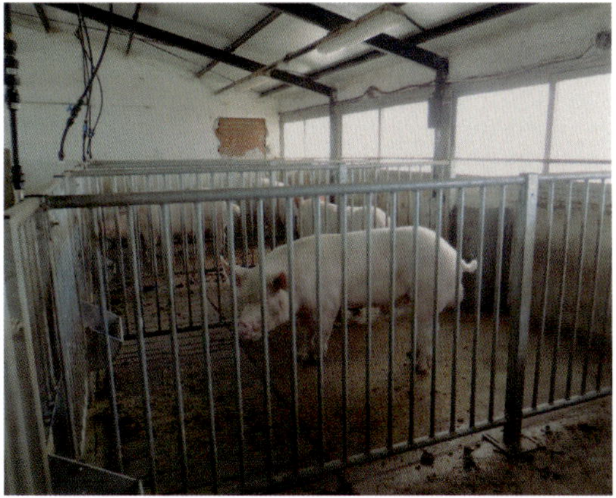

Figure 1. Individual boar enclosure, designed in accordance with European animal welfare standards (Directive 2001/88/EC, October 23, 2001). Consult United States Department of Agriculture (USDA), Animal Welfare Information Center (AWIC) and Animal Welfare Institute (AWI) for welfare standards in USA.

Collection area

The collection area should be designed so that the boar's attention is completely focused on the dummy sow, avoiding all other distractions. However, a safe area should also be available for the operator, in case any problems arise (Fig. 2). It is very important that the boar associates the semen collection room with a pleasant experience.

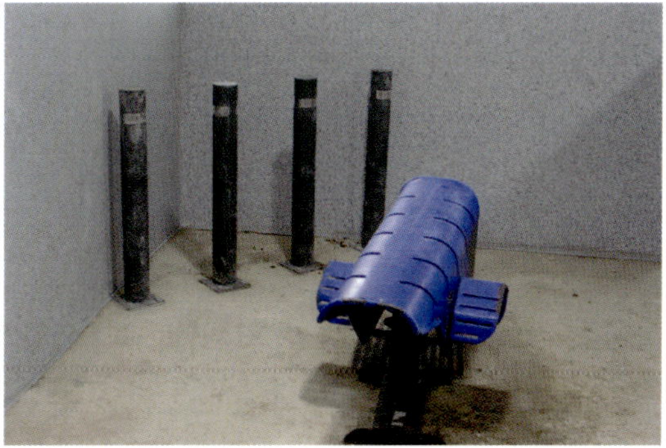

Figure 2. Collection room with a secure area for personnel.

Boar training

Training a boar requires patience, perseverance, and calm. It takes time for the boar to acclimate to the collection room. Not all boars behave in the same way, and stress should be avoided. Ideally, the personnel in charge should have some knowledge of the sexual behaviour of animals, in addition to patience and positivity.

During the training phase, the boar should be brought to the collection room 2 or 3 times a day at intervals of 15 to 20 minutes to acclimate to the dummy sow. He should be allowed time to inspect both the dummy sow and the room (Fig. 3).

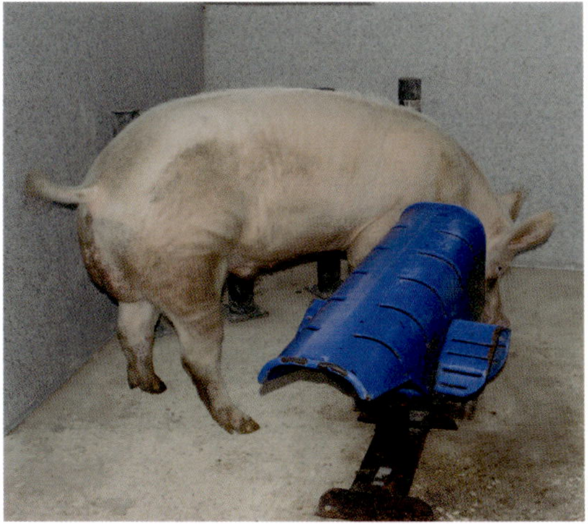

Figure 3. Boar inspecting the collection area.

Semen collection process

When the boar identifies the dummy sow, in many cases he will mount it naturally (Fig. 4), displaying a specific behaviour; sniffing, salivating, and striking the flanks of the dummy. It is sometimes advisable to impregnate the dummy sow with the semen of another boar (using the tapioca-like fraction), or with the urine of a sow in heat. The boar may also be stimulated with feed, but such practices should only be applied during the training phase.

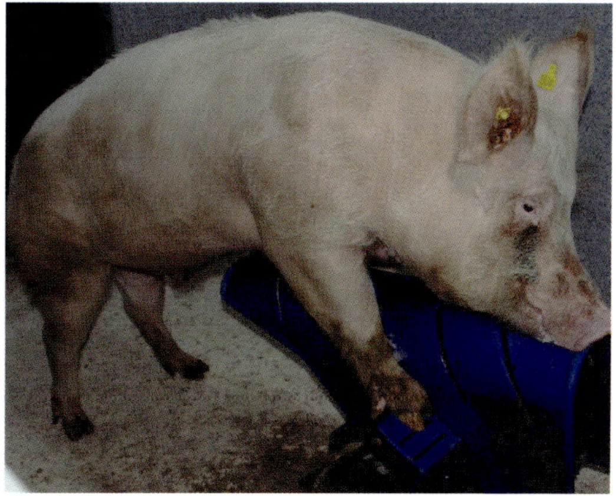

Figure 4. Boar mounting the dummy sow. Ensure that the dummy sow is at the appropriate height (specially for mounting by a young boar).

Once the boar has mounted the dummy sow, it is important to allow it to perform the copulatory pelvic thrusts. The foreskin should be massaged to stimulate the pelvic movements and exposure of the penis (Fig. 5). When the boar exposes its erect penis (Fig. 6) he should be approached from behind, without touching or scaring him, to begin the collection process.

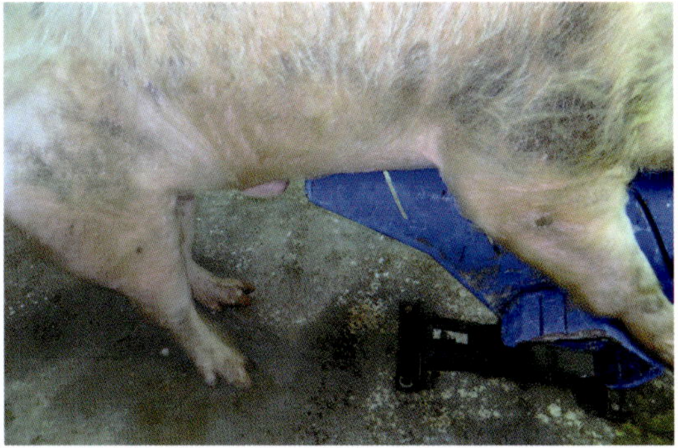

Figure 5. Once the boar has mounted the dummy sow, cleaning and massage of the foreskin must be carried out to stimulate extension of the penis.

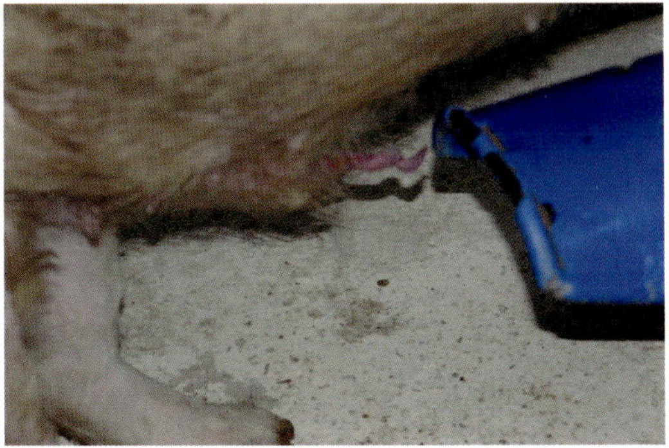

Figure 6. Male extending the penis.

After the boar has extended the penis, it is essential that uniform hand pressure is applied to the helical portion of the penis. It is important to exercise care at this moment, as pressure should not be applied either too close or too far from the distal portion of the penis (Figs. 7 and 8) (see Chapter 4).

The ideal age to start training is between 5 and 7 months. Caution should be used with young animals and semen should be collected once every seven days. In adult boars, the ejaculate is collected twice a week or, more precisely, 3 times at regular intervals over 2 weeks.

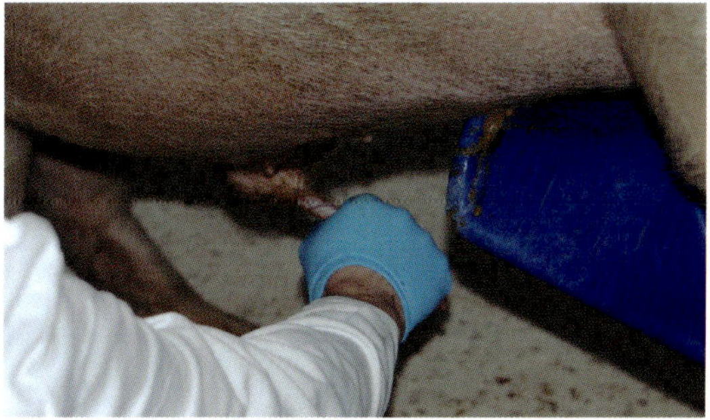

Figure 7. Application of uniform pressure to the penis.

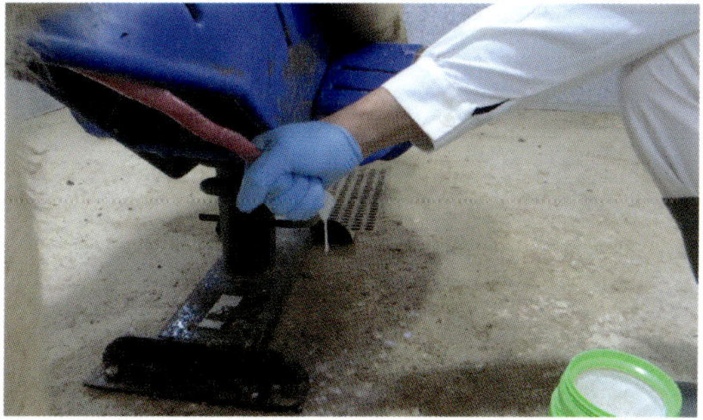

Figure 8. Erect boar penis. The boar begins the ejaculation process.

Regardless of the method used, the collection of semen must always meet the following conditions:

All materials and equipment that come into contact with the semen should be kept between 35 °C and 37 °C to avoid any shock (hot or cold).

Double glove technique

Semen should be obtained using techniques that minimise the possibility of contamination (Table 1).

Table 1. Factors influencing contamination of boar semen (adapted from Golderg et al., 2013).

Factors	Description
Boar hygiene	Clean: no noticeable dirt on the body of the boar Dirty: presence of dirt on the body
Preputial orifice hygiene	Clean: no noticeable dirt Dirty: presence of dirt
Preputial hair length	Short: <1 cm Long: ≥1 cm

Penis escapes during semen collection	Yes/ No
Dripping of preputial fluid from technician's hand	Into semen collection container Outside of semen collection container
Collection glove hygiene	Clean: has not touched anything other than the penis Dirty: has touched something other than the penis
Size of preputial diverticulum	Small:<6 cm Large: ≥6 cm
Inclination of semen collection container	Inclined: 45° during collection Not inclined: <45° during collection
Interval between entry of the technician into collecting room and mounting by the boar (min)	0–2 3–6 >6
Duration of semen collection (min)	2–5 6–7 >7
Age of boar (months)	8–18 >18

To collect semen, technicians should adhere to the following steps:

1. The hand that manipulates the foreskin should be covered with two vinyl gloves (one over the other).
2. The boar's foreskin should be emptied to remove its contents, as well as any remaining urine that could contaminate the ejaculate. The preputial orifice is massaged with gauze soaked in antiseptic and disinfectant (highly diluted to avoid damaging the mucous membranes). This massaging of the foreskin stimulates pelvic movement and the expulsion of preputial fluid. The boar will be stimulated and externalise the penis.
3. At this precise moment the first glove, which has been in contact with the foreskin, is removed.
4. Next, the hand should be closed, allowing the penis to pass through 4 or 5 times. The placement of the hand and the strong pressure exerted on the boar's spiral-shaped penis mimics the morphology of the uterus of a sow in heat (Figs. 1 and 2). When the penis is held firmly, the boar begins to ejaculate (Figs. 3 and 4).
5. The penis must be held as horizontal as possible to prevent contamination of the ejaculate with traces of urine.

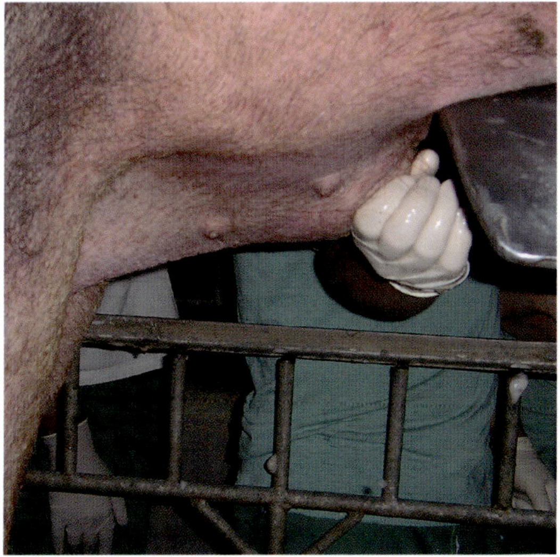

Figure 1. Close hand around the penis, allowing the penis to pass through the hand several times when pelvic movement begins.

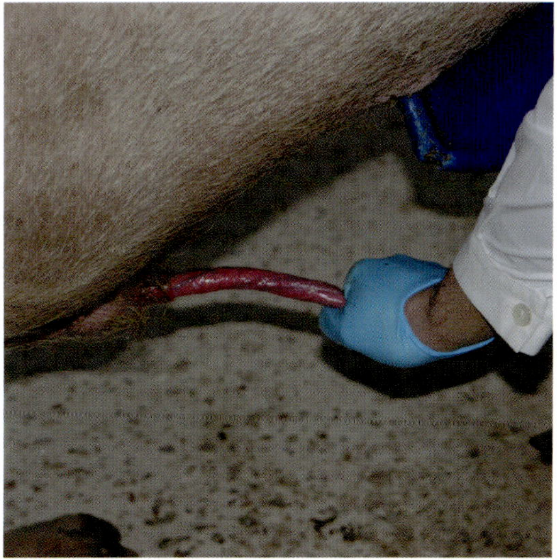

Figure 2. The firm pressure exerted upon the penis stimulates ejaculation.

The pressure the technician will need to exert upon the penis can vary depending on the boar. Be sure to exert the correct pressure upon the penis; failure to do so can have a negative effect on the boar, which will then retract the penis and refuse to mount the dummy.

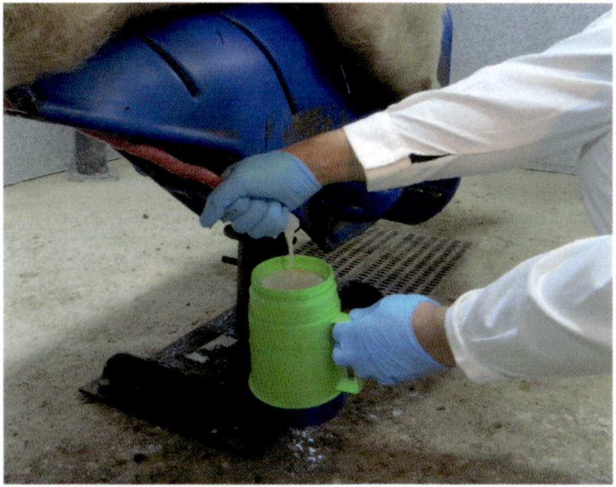

Figure 3. Moment of ejaculation.

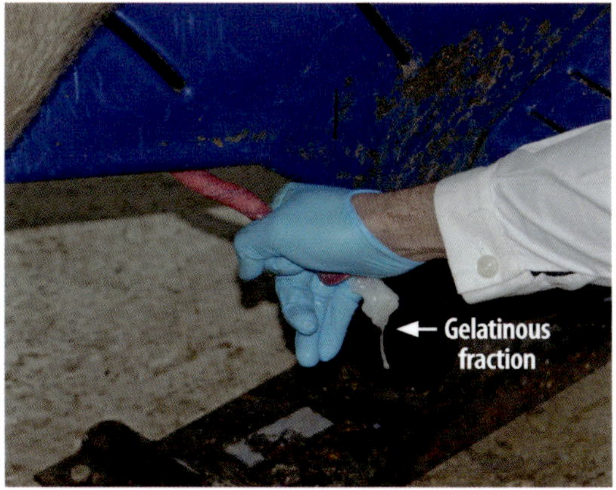

Figure 4. Position of the penis in the technician's hand.

The whole process of collection takes between 5 and 10 minutes.

The length of the preputial hair should be checked every 15 to 30 days, and the hair trimmed if necessary to prevent contamination of the ejaculate (Fig. 5).

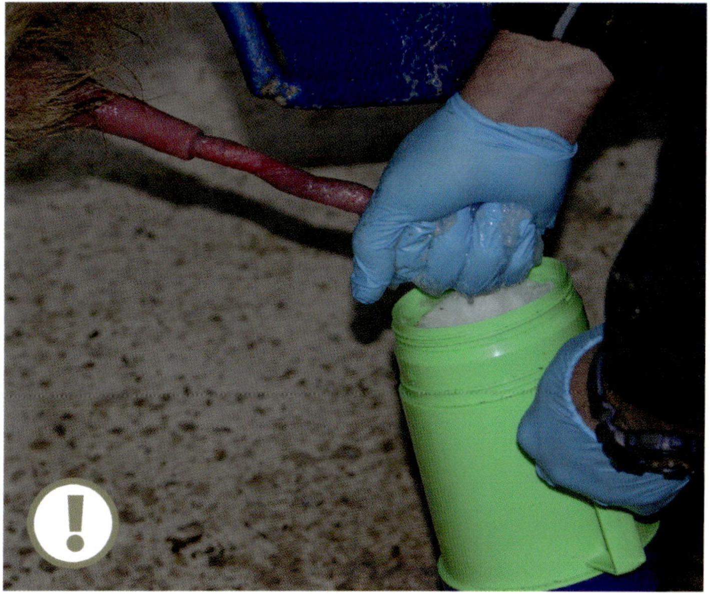

Figure 5. The preputial hair is longer than 1 cm and should be trimmed.

It is very important to minimise the possibility of contamination during the semen collection process (Figs. 6-9).

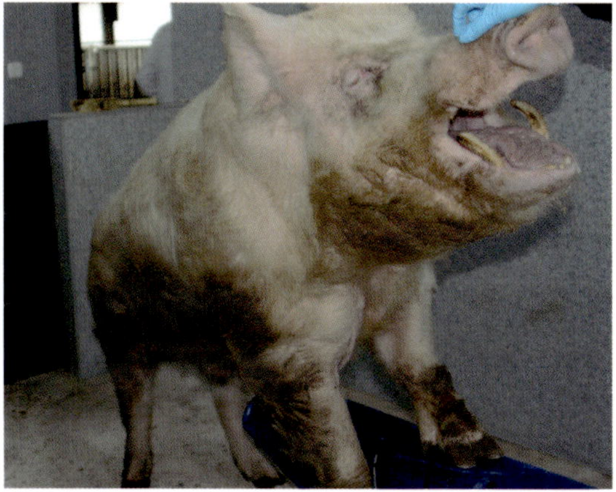

Figure 6. Dirt on the body of the boar increases the likelihood of contamination of the ejaculate.

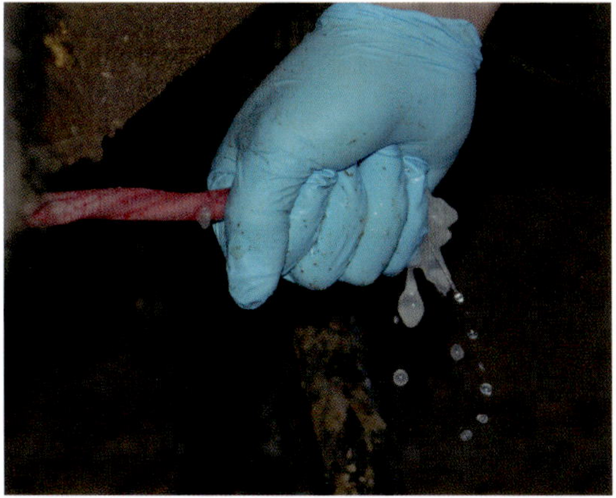

Figure 7. The penis must remain as horizontal as possible to avoid contamination of the ejaculate with urine.

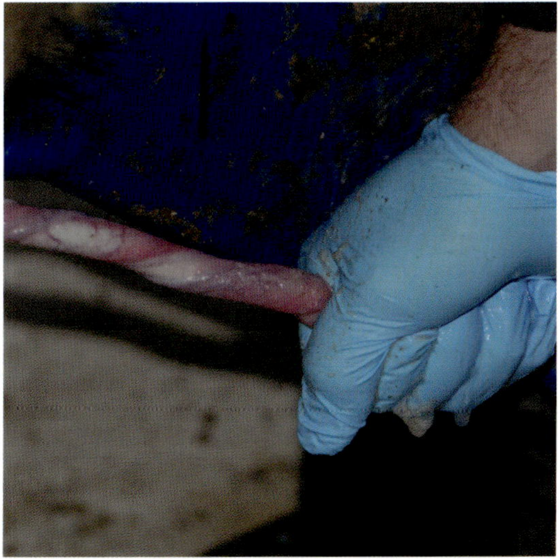

Figure 8. If the dummy is dirty, it can stain the glove, thus contaminating the ejaculate.

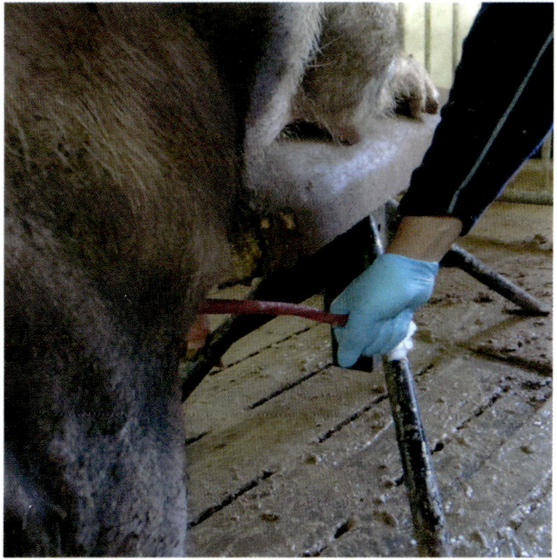

Figure 9. Dirty floor in collection room. Contamination of the ejaculate is more likely in these conditions.

Sperm fractions

Boar ejaculate consists of sperm and secretions produced by the accessory glands (seminal vesicles, prostate, and Cowper's glands). These fluids can be classified into several fractions with distinct characteristics (Table 2). The first fraction of boar ejaculate is the pre-sperm fraction. It is transparent, with a volume of 10–15 ml, and is usually heavily contaminated. It contains no sperm.

The pre-sperm fraction should not be collected.

Table 2. Characteristics of the sperm fractions of the boar.

Characteristic	Pre-sperm fraction	Sperm fraction	Post-sperm fraction
Volume	10–15 ml	100 ml	200 ml
% sperm	0	90	10
Colour	Transparent	White	Grey-white
Density	Clear fluid	Creamy white	Clear fluid

The second fraction is the sperm-rich fraction (Figs. 10 and 11). This fraction (50–100 ml) contains the highest concentration of sperm. It is dense, white, and has a milky appearance. This fraction is collected using a filter to separate it from the gelatinous material known as "tapioca" (Figs. 12 and 13) produced by the bulbourethral or Cowper's glands.

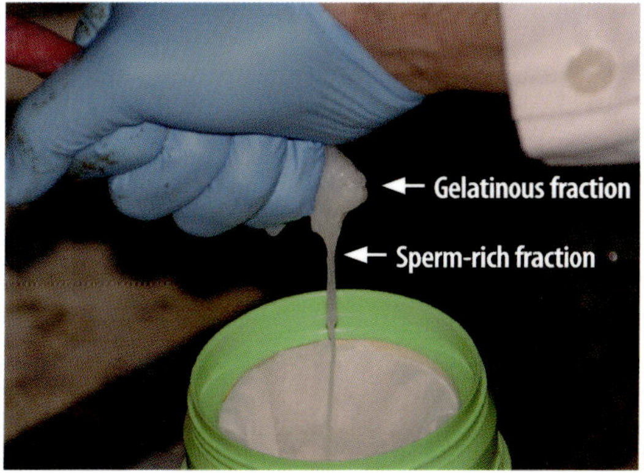

Figure 10. The fraction to be retained can be identified by colour.

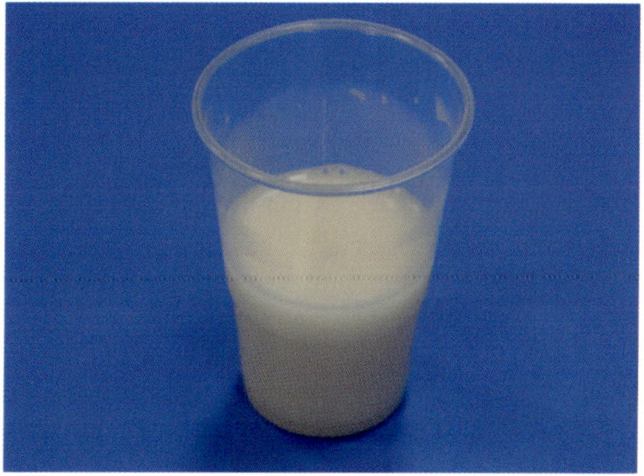

Figure 11. Fraction with highest sperm content (sperm-rich fraction).

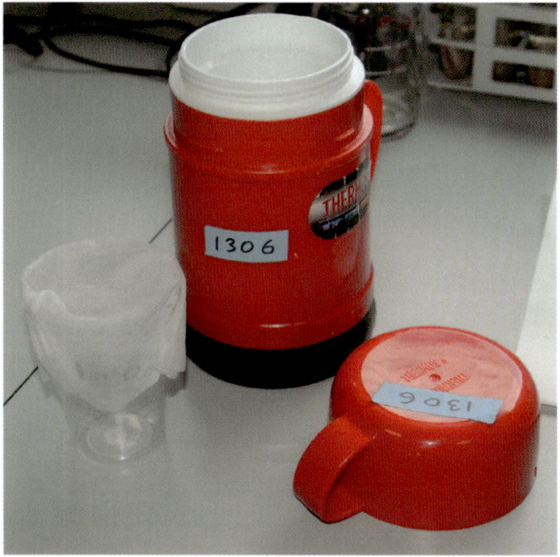

Figure 12. Flask and collection receptacle with gauze or filter to separate the tapioca.

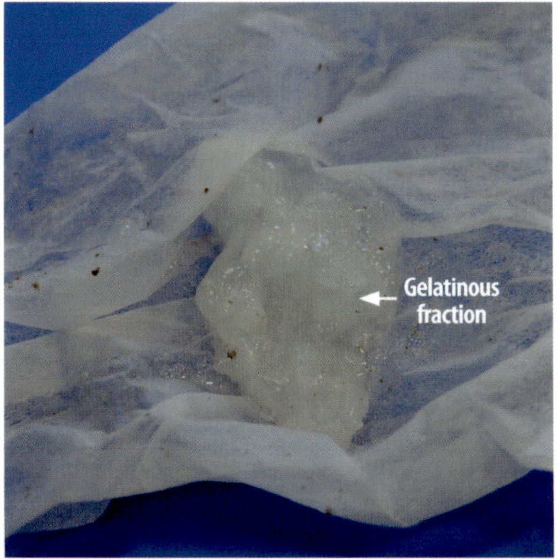

Figure 13. Appearance of tapioca.

Collection of gelatinous fraction is not recommended. It can be separated using a filter (Fig. 14).

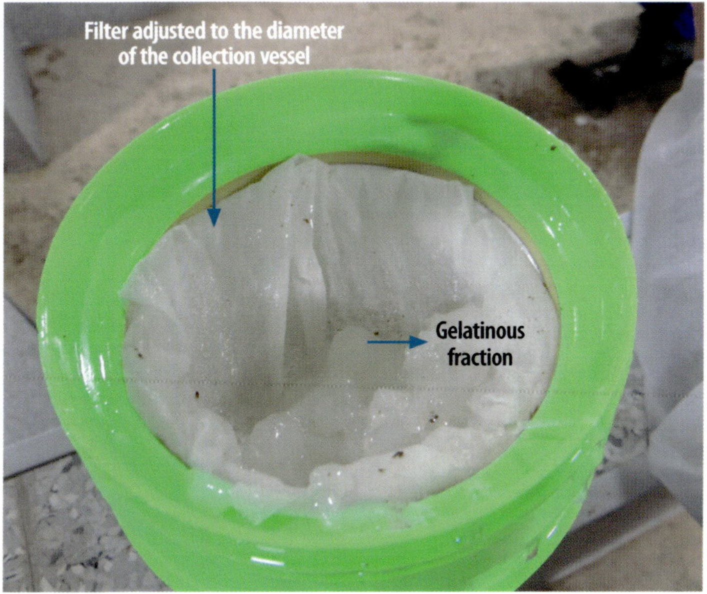

Figure 14. Detail of filter.

The third fraction (Figs. 15 and 16), of about 150–200 ml, consists of secretions of the accessory glands and contains little sperm. This fraction is grey-white, and contains many gelatinous lumps, which in nature form a plug in the cervix to prevent backflow of the ejaculate. This fraction should not be collected as it can promote agglutination of the sperm.

In young boars it can be difficult to distinguish these three phases, and extra care is required during the collection process. However, in adult boars these three phases can be clearly distinguished.

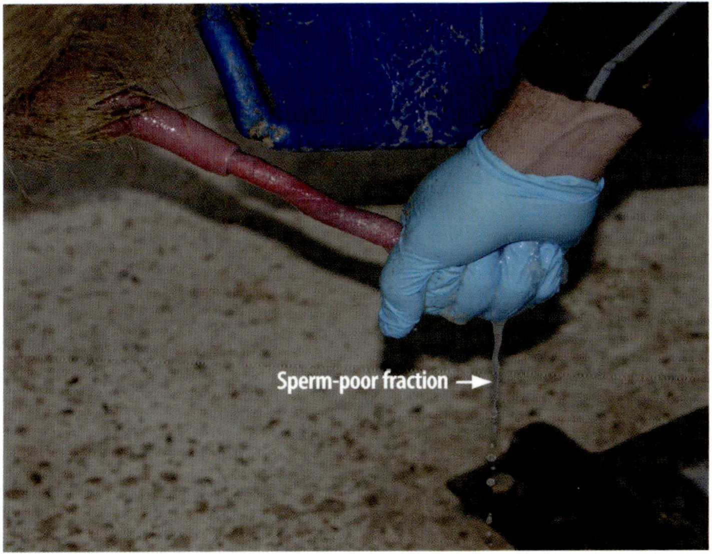

Figure 15. Sperm-poor fraction (transparent colour).

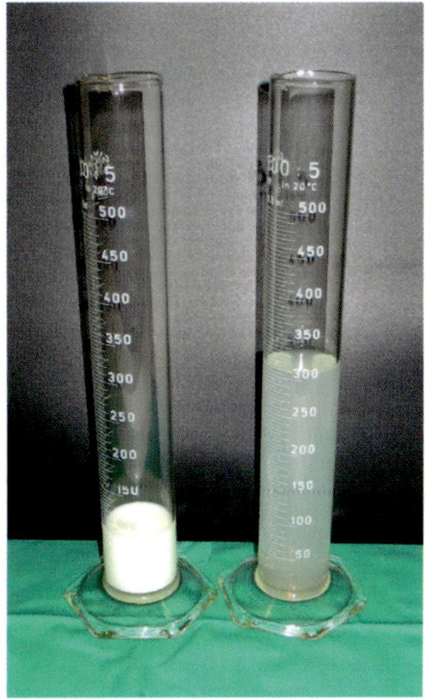

Figure 16. Comparison of sperm-rich fraction (80 ml) and post-sperm fraction (320 ml).

5 Evaluation of semen quality

Introduction

Semen quality is mainly dependent on factors associated with the boar (age, genetics, and health status) and with the procedures used to collect and store ejaculate. Similarly, seminal characteristics may change depending on the conditions under which the ejaculate is collected and the time elapsed since collection.

The doses used for AI are selected based on two parameters:

1. Quality, defined by the motility and morphology of the sperm, the functional integrity of the acrosomal membrane, and the absence of microbial contamination.

2. Sperm concentration, determined by number of sperm.

Good quality boar semen is essential to obtain optimal fertility on the farm. The routine tests currently used to assess semen quality include evaluation of sperm motility, morphology, and concentration.

It is also imperative to maintain stable conditions when handling ejaculate in the laboratory, avoiding variations in temperature, osmolarity, and/or pH, which can alter the initial characteristics of ejaculate and result in outcomes far below the reproductive targets of the farm.

Semen quality control methods can vary depending on where they are conducted: on the farm, in an AI facility, or in a specialised laboratory. In any case, the following describes the evaluation of macroscopic and microscopic semen parameters.

Volume

The volume of the ejaculate can be determined using a warm (35–37 °C) graduated cylinder, or by weighing on a precision scales, assuming that one gram corresponds to a volume of one cubic centimetre or millilitre (Fig. 1). The volume of the sperm-rich fraction is between 80 ml and 150 ml.

A larger volume of ejaculate does not imply a higher number of sperm. This parameter is evaluated to determine the number of seminal doses.

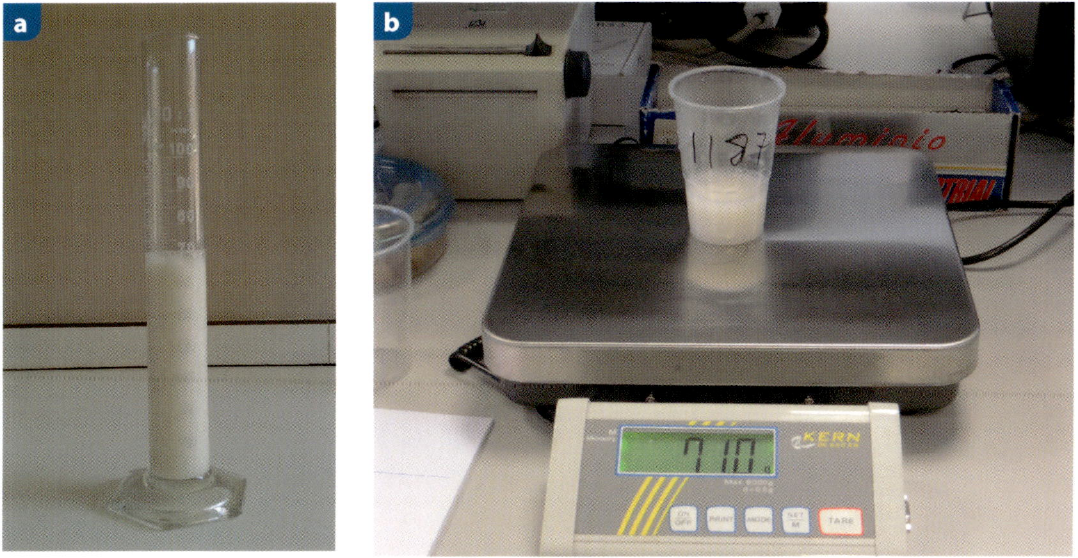

Figure 1. Determination of ejaculate volume using a graduated cylinder (a) or a precision balance (b).

Motility

Determination of motility is a crucial aspect of routine semen quality control. The progressive motility of sperm is an indicator of good metabolic status and the presence of intact membranes.

On the farm, estimation of the percentage of motile sperm is performed using an optical light microscope. A small drop of fresh semen is placed on a heated (37 °C) slide and covered with a coverslip. The sample should be thin enough to allow observation of the movement of each sperm. The type of movement exhibited by sperm is related to the quality thereof, and is evaluated on a scale of 0 to 5 (Fig. 2).

The results obtained using this technique depend on the experience of the evaluator. Therefore, the process of preparing the sample (the dilution, the type of diluent, temperature, etc.) should be standardised to reduce the error between estimates for each of the different samples analysed.

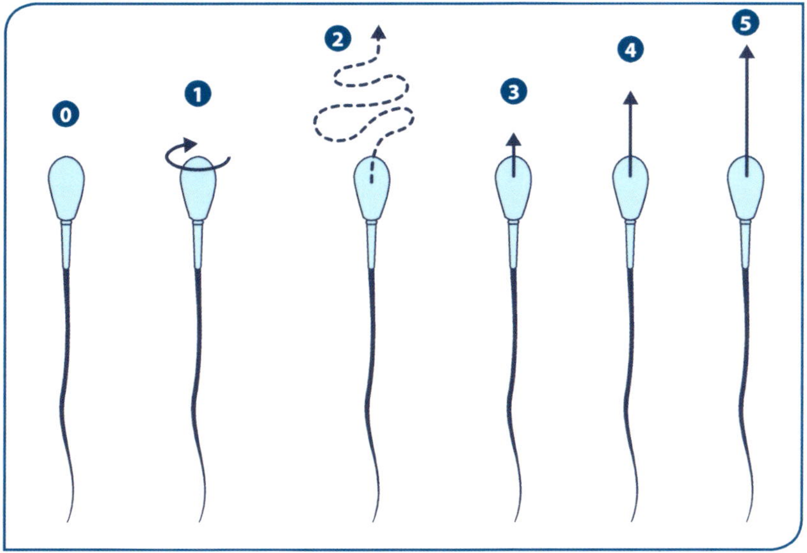

0. Immobile sperm.

1. Sperm showing little movement; the head remains fixed and only the tail remains in motion.

2. Sperm moving in circles, with some progressive movement.

3. Sperm showing progressive and sinuous movement.

4. Sperm showing progressive and rapid movement.

5. Sperm showing very fast progressive movement.

Figure 2. Scale of 0 to 5 for the assessment of sperm motility.

In the last 20 years, motility assessment has been improved by the use of specialised software, such as the Computer-Assisted Semen Analysis System (CASA). This system provides very accurate individual information about the speed and morphology of sperm, as well as the extent and type of movement, thus providing more objective information on the aforementioned parameters (Verstegen et al., 2001).

Motility assessment should be performed daily once stored samples have been appropriately diluted.

Freshly obtained boar semen should contain a high percentage of mobile sperm (minimum 70 %) with a movement score of at least 3.

Morphology (abnormalities)

Boars used in AI programs should have a low percentage of abnormally shaped sperm.

A large number of morphologically abnormal sperm is indicative of alterations during sperm development or maturation, or incorrect semen processing.

Abnormalities include loose heads, folded (whip-like) or coiled (balled) tails, broken tails, and double heads or tails. Overuse of boars results in an increase in the number of immature sperm, which can be identified by the presence of cytoplasmic droplets in the intermediate tract (Fig. 3). These droplets are remnants of cytoplasm that remain after spermatogenesis and are located in the intermediate tract. Cytoplasmic droplets (proximal or distal) are generally the most common morphological alteration. Febrile processes may increase the number of folded tails. Improper handling of the ejaculate (thermal or osmotic shock) may cause an increase in the number of sperm with folded tails.

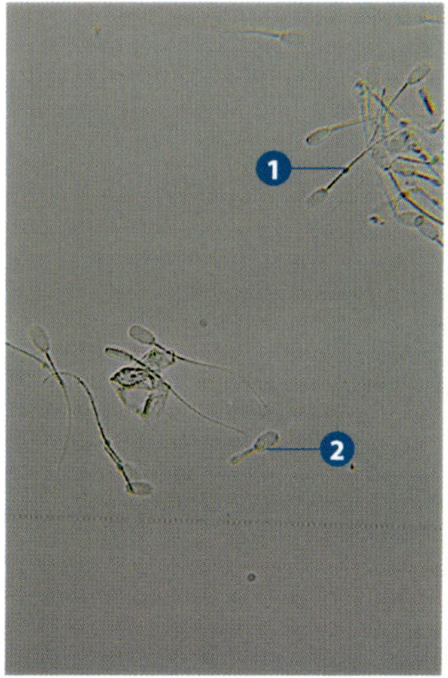

Figure 3. Sperm containing a distal cytoplasmic droplet (1) and sperm with a folded (whip-like) tail (2) (40×).

The total percentage of cytoplasmic droplets in ejaculate used for AI should not exceed 15 %, especially if refrigerated semen is used. Other alterations should not exceed 5 %, such that the total percentage of morphological alterations is less than 20 %.

Ejaculate used for AI should contain 80 % morphologically normal sperm. Folded tails are more significant than the presence of cytoplasmic droplets. Semen in which more than 40 % of the sperm have folded tails should not be used for AI.

Figure 4 shows the position of the cytoplasmic droplet and the types of tail alterations most commonly seen in boar semen.

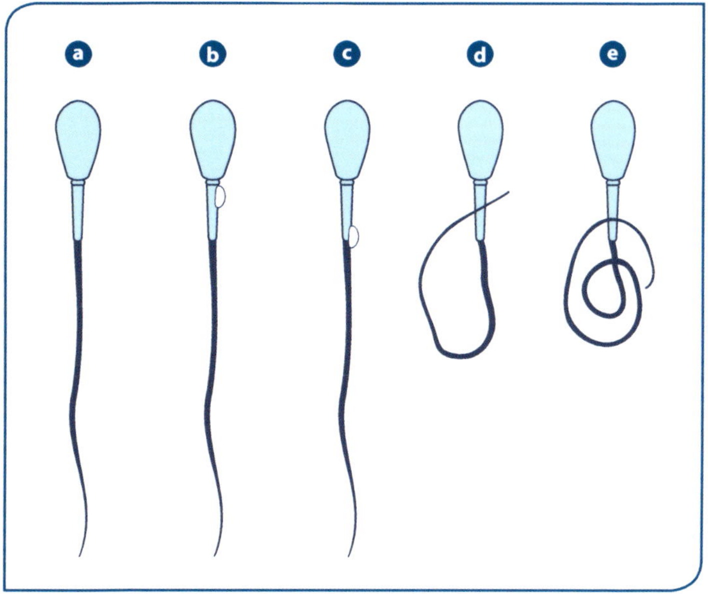

Figure 4. Normal sperm and common morphological alterations in boar sperm. Normal (a), proximal cytoplasmic droplet (b), cytoplasmic droplet at the end of the intermediate tract (c), folded tail (whip-like) (d), and coiled (balled) tail (e).

Normally an optical microscope with phase contrast is used to observe semen samples fixed in 3 % formalin-citrate solution (Fig. 5).

Several stains for the analysis of sperm morphology in dry preparations are commercially available (e.g. eosin-nigrosin).

The percentage of normal sperm can be calculated using a Bürker chamber (see next section). This calculation requires the analysis of 200 to 400 sperm and is performed at the same time that the assessment of sperm morphology.

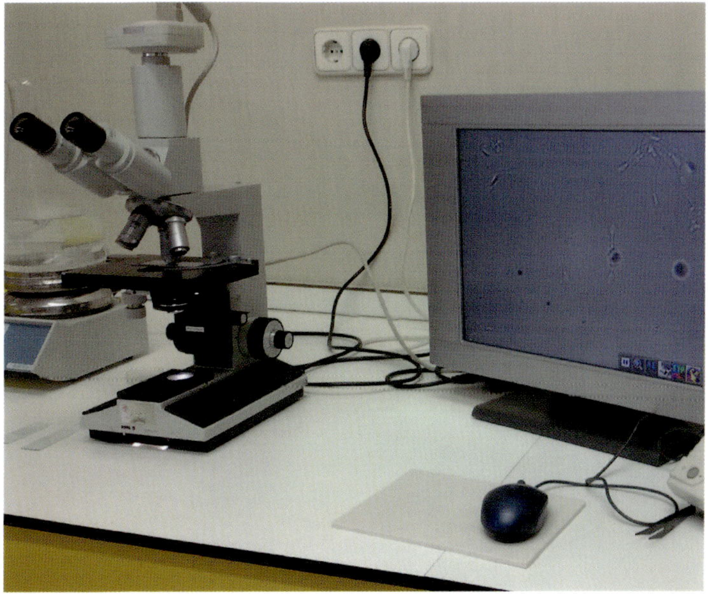

Figure 5. Phase contrast microscopy.

Sperm concentration and sperm count

In AI, the objective is to keep highly fertile sperm viable for a long period, and to use the minimum concentration of sperm per dose.

Evaluating sperm concentration is part of the routine analysis carried out to assess ejaculate quality. On a farm, this is achieved using a cell counting chamber (Figs. 6-8), whereas in AI facilities automated systems are used.

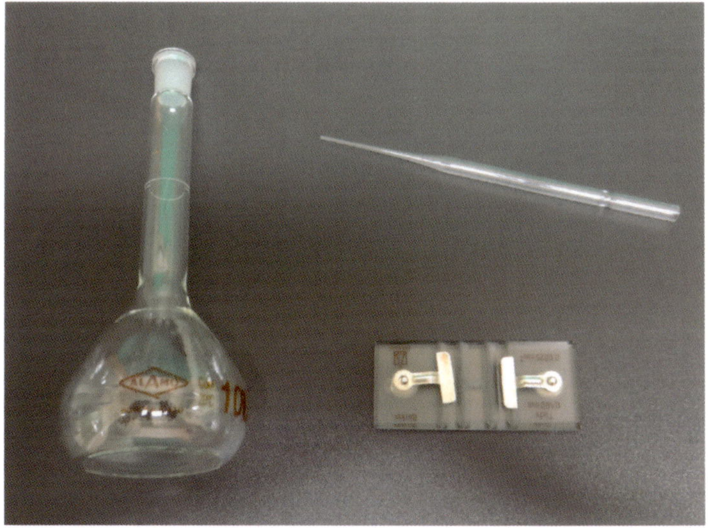

Figure 6. Materials required to determine sperm count: flask, pipette, and cell counting chamber.

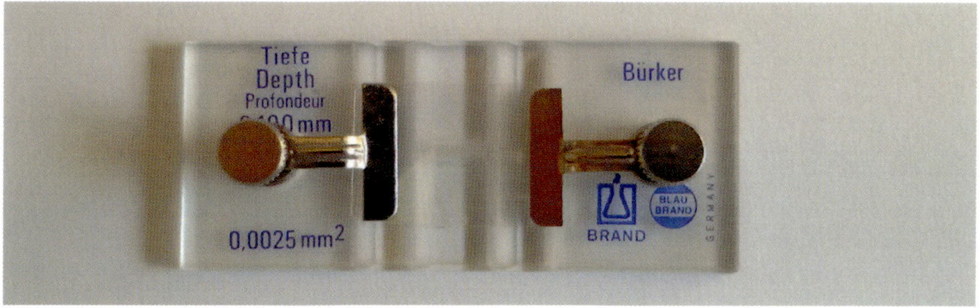

Figure 7. Bürker chamber used to determine sperm count.

The sperm concentration (no. of sperm/ml) is calculated using the following formula:

Number of viable sperm counted in 40 squares × dilution factor (1:100) × volume of Bürker chamber

⇓

e.g. $52 \times 100 \times 10^5$

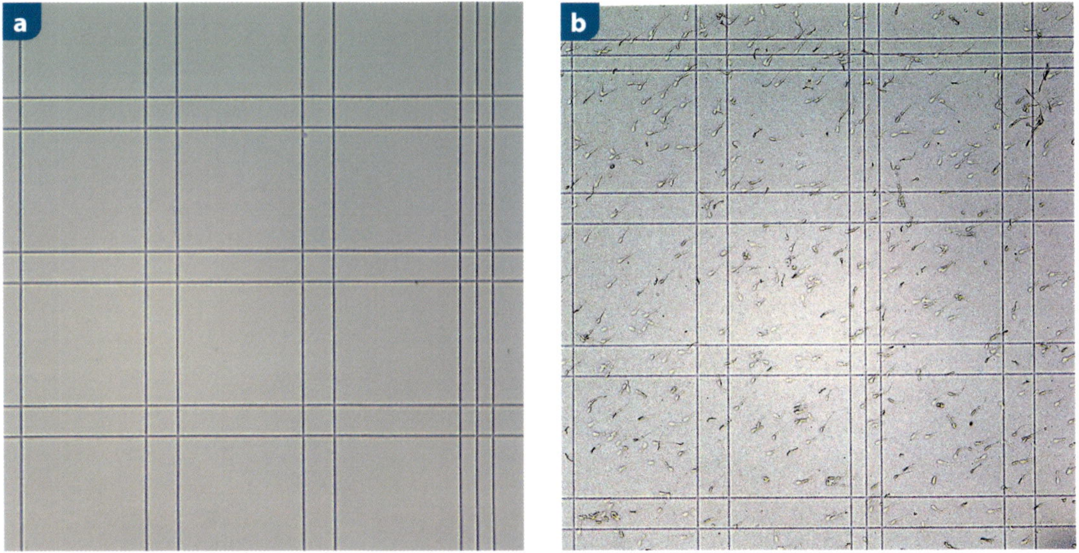

Figure 8. Bürker chamber. Empty (a) and loaded with a semen sample (b).

Total number of sperm present in ejaculate

Due to the large number of samples to be analysed every day in an AI facility, sperm concentration is calculated using a photocolorimeter or automated counting systems such as photometers (single wavelength) or spectrophotometers (multiple wavelengths). These methods, which use commercial computerised analysis software, are faster than the cell-counting chamber method (Hansen et al., 2006), but also have some drawbacks. Here, we describe the manual counting method.

To calculate the total number of sperm, simply multiply the volume of ejaculate by its concentration (Figs. 9-11). In the example, in 125 ml of ejaculate collected:

$125 \times 52 \times 10^7 = 6{,}500 \times 10^7$ total sperm in the ejaculate (i.e. $6{,}500 \times 10^7$ viable sperm in 125 ml of ejaculate).

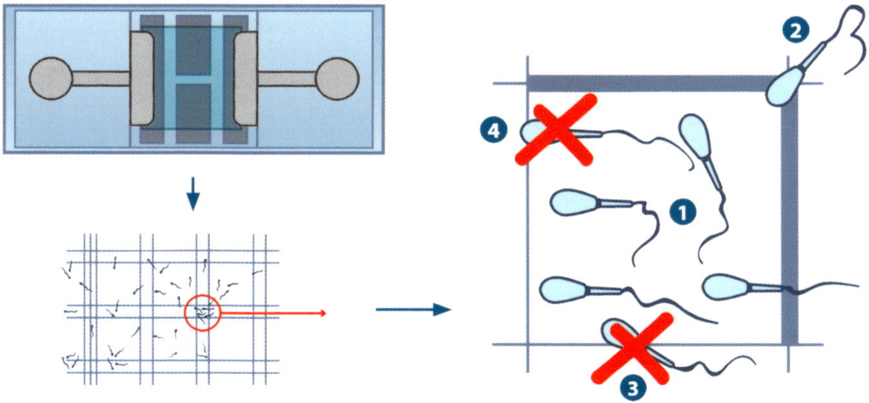

Figure 9. Schematic showing grid arrangement in Bürker chamber and sperm to be counted (left). Example of counting sperm in one of the 40 squares (right). The following sperm are considered valid: those with heads inside the square (1) and those outside of the square but whose heads touch two sides (the top and right sides) (2). Sperm that are inside or outside the square but touch the finer sides of the square (bottom and left), are not counted (3 and 4). In this example there are five valid sperm.

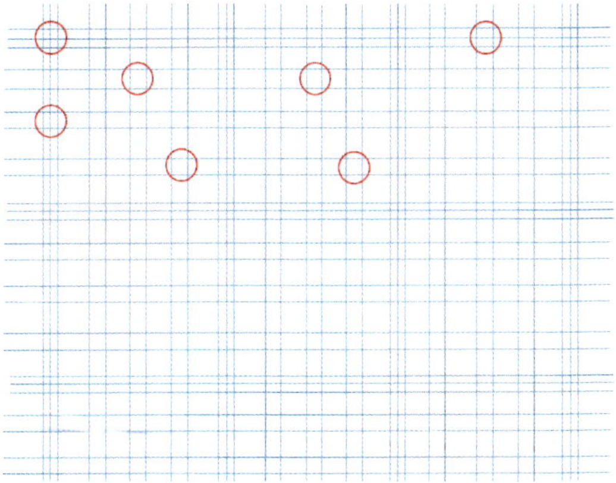

Figure 10. Detail of the chamber, which consists of 369 small squares of 0.0025 mm^2 each. It is only necessary to count 40 squares (examples indicated in red).

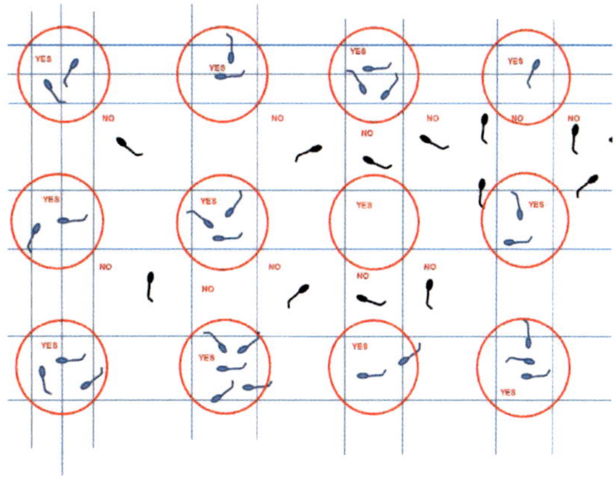

Figure 11. Counting system for Bürker chamber. Counting begins at the beginning of the first row. Each row contains 13 squares, which should be counted using a zigzag counting technique. Counting is performed from left to right. When the row is finished, drop to the row below and count from right to left. Continue until 40 squares have been counted.

Estimation of the number of abnormal sperm is performed while determining the concentration (Figs. 12 and 13). This takes approximately five minutes per semen sample.

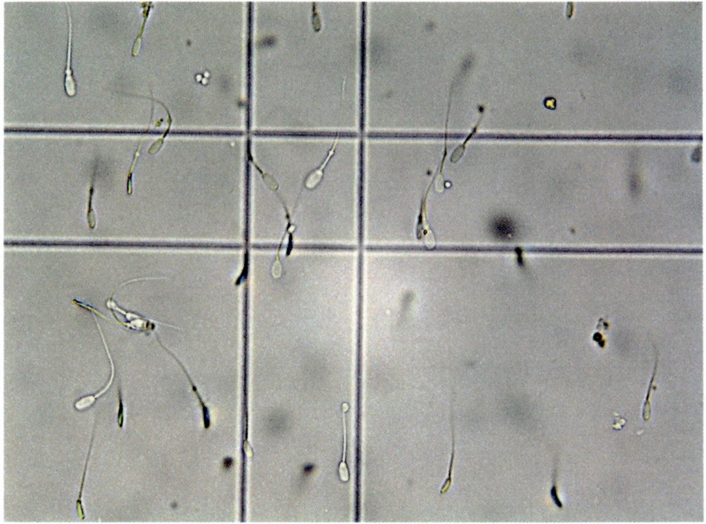

Figure 12. Bürker chamber (40×). In this example only two sperm with a distal droplet should be recorded (central small square).

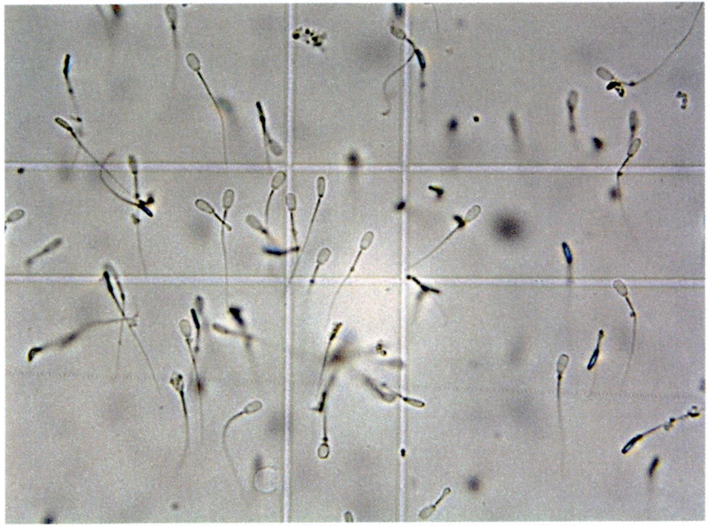

Figure 13. Bürker chamber (40×). Three sperm should be recorded in this example; one normal and two with distal cytoplasmic droplets (central small square).

Acrosome morphology

The acrosome is located at the apical end of the sperm head, and contains a series of enzymes necessary for the fertilisation process. Evaluating acrosome integrity is a routine technique in specialised laboratories, and requires a phase contrast microscope. The acrosome is categorised following the classification system of Pursel and Johnson (1975), as shown in Figure 14 and described below:

- Normal apical ridge (NAR): the acrosome is fully adhered to the nucleus of the sperm, with a clear boundary between the two and with a distinct crescent shape at the apical ridge of the head (Figs. 14a and 15).
- Normal apical ridge with particles (NAR'): as described for NAR, except for the presence of small adherent particles in the apical region and in the postnuclear area of the acrosome (Fig. 14b).
- Damaged apical ridge (DAR): sperm are identified by the presence of particles in the area posterior to the apical ridge of the acrosome (damaged), which lends them an irregular shape (Fig. 14c).
- Missing apical ridge (MAR): sperm have lost the apical ridge, but part of the acrosome remains firmly attached to the head (Figs. 14d, 16, and 18).
- Loose acrosomal cap (LAC): characterised by the formation of vesicles in the anterior part of the acrosome (Figs. 14e, 16, and 17).

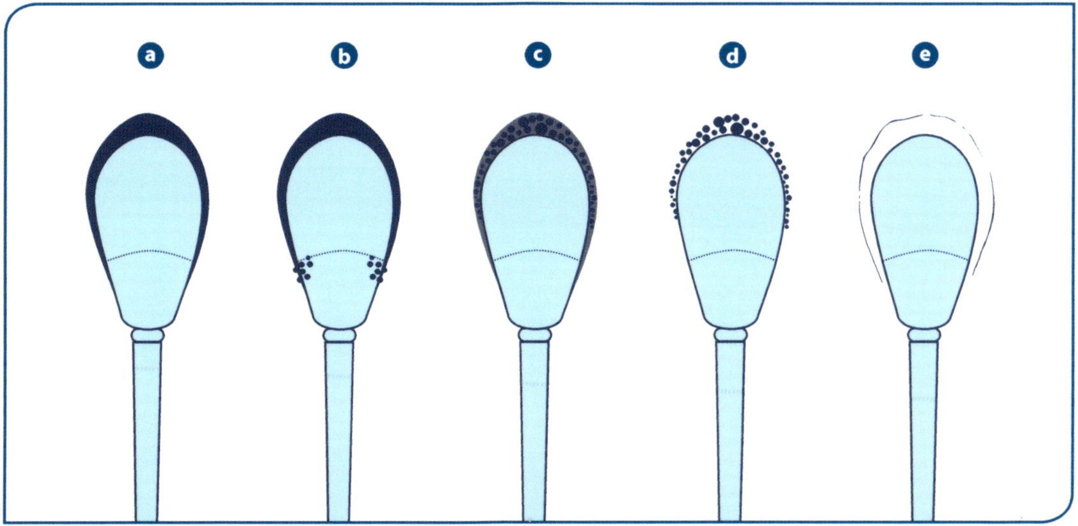

Figure 14. Categorisation of acrosome integrity: normal apical ridge (NAR) (a), normal apical ridge with particles (NAR') (b), damaged apical ridge (DAR) (c), missing apical ridge (MAR) (d), and loose acrosomal cap (LAC) (e).

In routine analyses, only normal acrosomes are counted. Sperm exhibiting damage to the acrosome are included in the acrosomal damage category (without specifying the extent of the alteration).

Ejaculates accepted for AI must contain between 85 % and 90 % NAR sperm.

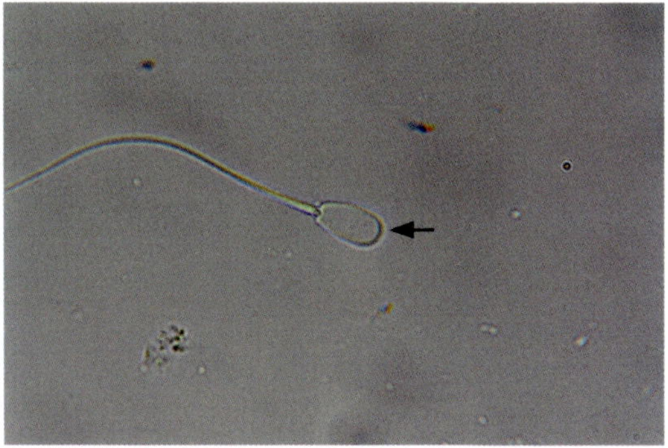

Figure 15. NAR sperm, with an intact apical ridge and a perfectly adhered acrosome, indicated with arrow (100×).

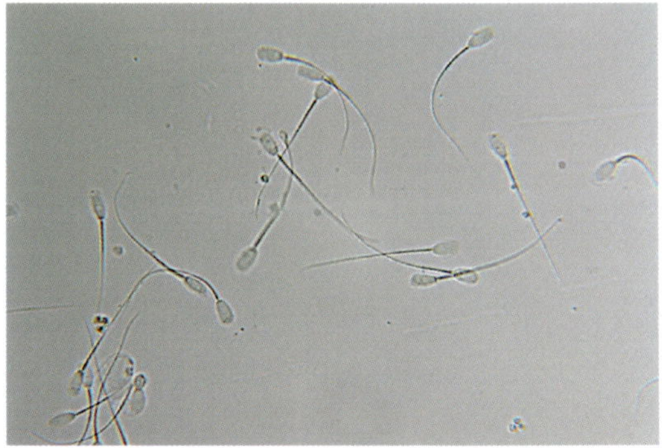

Figure 16. Sperm with a missing apical ridge (MAR) and loose acrosome caps (LAC) (40×).

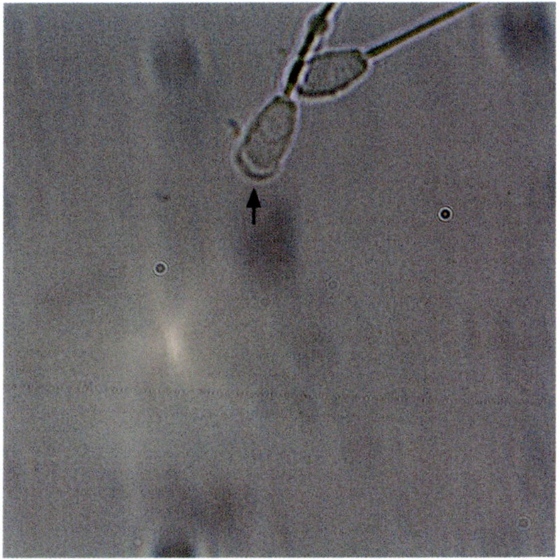

Figure 17. Detail of a sperm with loose acrosomal cap (LAC), indicated with arrow (100×).

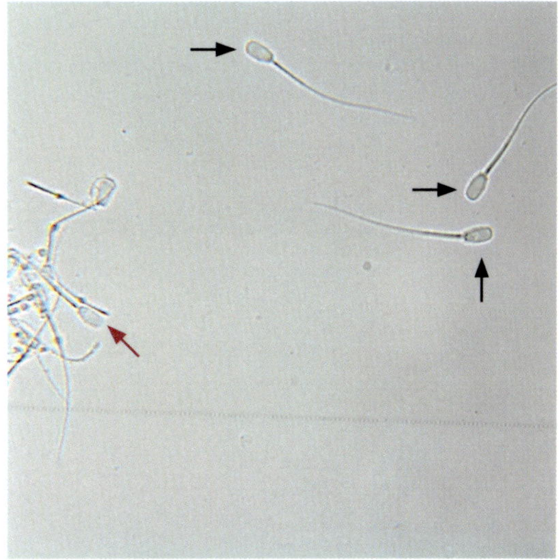

Figure 18. NAR sperm, with normal apical ridges (black arrows) and MAR sperm with missing apical ridge (red arrow) (40×).

Agglutination

The agglutination process (Fig. 19) reduces the number of sperm available for fertilisation and can be caused by several factors:

- Inappropriate semen collection methods, which result in the presence of gelatine in the ejaculate, or poor sanitary conditions.
- Pathological processes of the boar that increase desquamation of epithelial cells (Fig. 20).
- Increasing temperatures, which can also enhance agglutination.

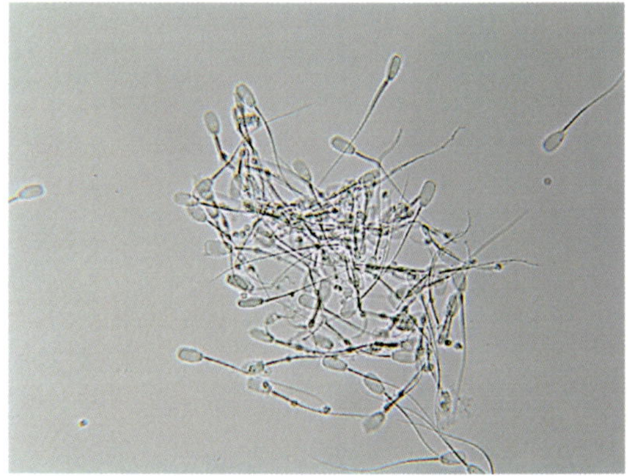

Figure 19. Sperm that have agglutinated due to interactions between one another (40×).

- Treatments received by boars (both preventive and curative) can result in temporary alterations in ejaculate quality, and thus should be taken into account.

The estimated degree of agglutination is represented by plus signs as follows: +, mild clumping (Fig. 21); ++, moderate clumping; +++, severe clumping (Fig. 22).

In some cases, depending on the boar or due to a temperature increase (e.g. during the summer), it is recommended to add about 50 ml of diluent to the collection flask to reduce agglutination. This can somewhat attenuate the adverse effects of agglutination.

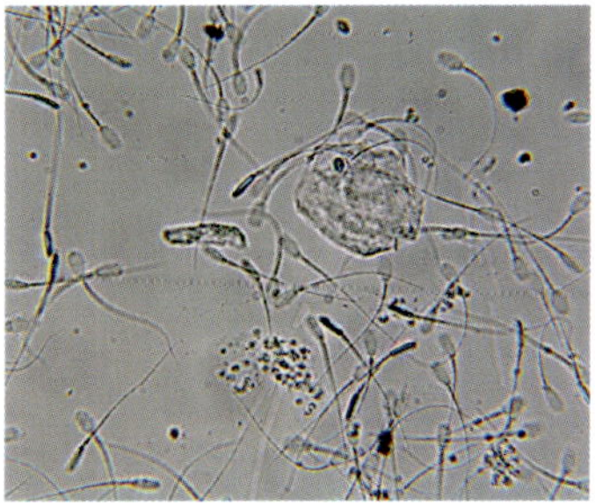

Figure 20. Sperm that have agglutinated due to the presence of cells, the result of epithelial desquamation (40×).

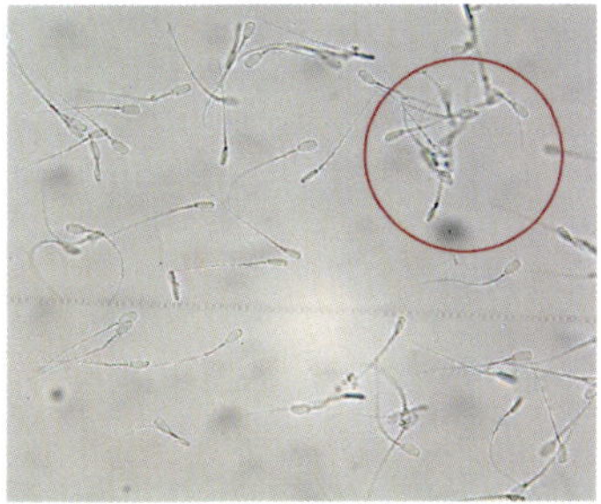

Figure 21. Mild clumping. There is only one group of sperm in the field. (40×). Estimated degree of agglutination: +.

Figure 22. Severe clumping. Most of the sperm are agglutinated (10×). Estimated degree of agglutination: +++.

Data sheet for monitoring boars

Both in AI facilities and on farms, it is important to create a data sheet for each boar, in which each of the aforementioned parameters is recorded.

Table 1 shows an example of a data sheet used to record semen collection from each boar, including the rate of collection, the various parameters that determine the quality of the ejaculate, and the number of doses processed.

Table 1. Example of a data sheet for individual monitoring of boars.

Boar No.:					**Breed:**							
Date	Volume (sperm-rich fraction)	Concentration (Sp/ml)	Motility (%)	Normal acrosomes (%)	Abnormal forms (%)			Agglutination			No. of doses	Observations
					PD	DD	C	+	++	+++		

Abnormal forms. PD: proximal droplet; DD: distal droplet; C: folded tail; Sp: sperm.

Agglutination. (+): mild; (++): moderate; (+++): severe.

Semen extenders

Semen extenders are liquid diluents added to the ejaculate to maintain its fertilising capacity for a period of 24 hours to 7 days depending on the type of extender used; this solution is stored at 15 °C. Semen extenders contain essential elements (ions, energy, antibiotics, etc.) and the necessary conditions (pH buffering capacity, etc.) to maintain the stability of the structural (membrane) and functional (metabolism) characteristics of the spermatozoa (Table 1).

Table 1. Composition of boar semen extenders used commercially in the preparation of refrigerated semen doses (all contain antibiotics, although this is not indicated in the table).

Component (g/l)	Short-term extender (1–3 days)			Long-term extender (>4 days)
	BTS	KIEV	IVT	ZORLESCO
Glucose	37.0	60.0	3.0	11.5
EDTA	1.25	3.7	-	2.3
Sodium-citrate	6.0	3.7	24.3	11.7
Sodium-bicarbonate	1.25	1.2	2.4	1.25
Potassium chloride	0.75	-	0.4	-
Tris	-	-	-	6.5
Citric acid	-	-	-	4.1
Cysteine	-	-	0.05[1]	0.1
BSA	-	-	-	5.0

[1] Acetylcysteine. Modified from Johnson et al., 2000.

Extender preparation

Extender preparation involves dissolution of the components in powder form in a flask of distilled water, and subsequent homogenisation for 15 to 30 minutes. In some cases a dye is added to ensure that all the required ingredients have been included (Fig. 1). It is essential to carry out biological and physico-chemical controls to check water quality. Ready-to-use porcine extenders are also commercially available. As soon as the number of doses is determined and the required volume of extender established, the final dilution is prepared. This should be done within 15 minutes of semen collection.

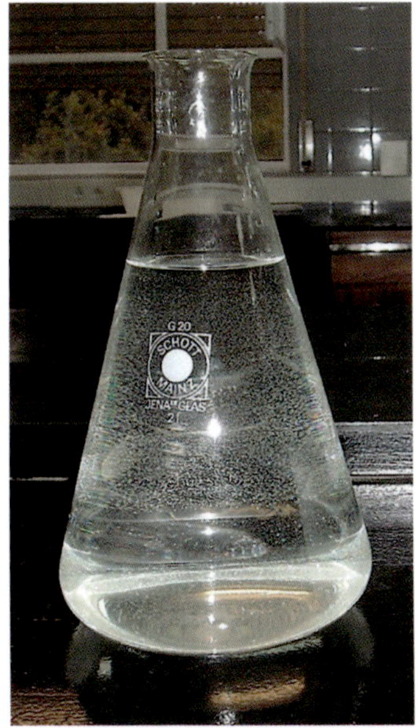

Figure 1. Erlenmeyer flask containing extender and distilled water.

The ejaculate and extender must be at the same temperature. This can be achieved using a water bath set at 37 °C (Figs. 2 and 3).

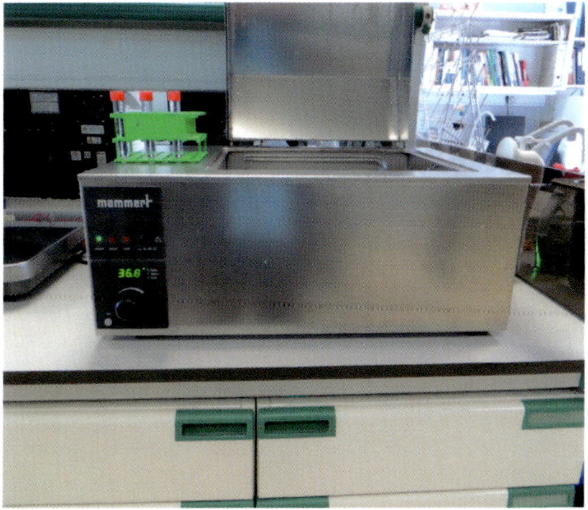

Figure 2. Water bath (37 °C).

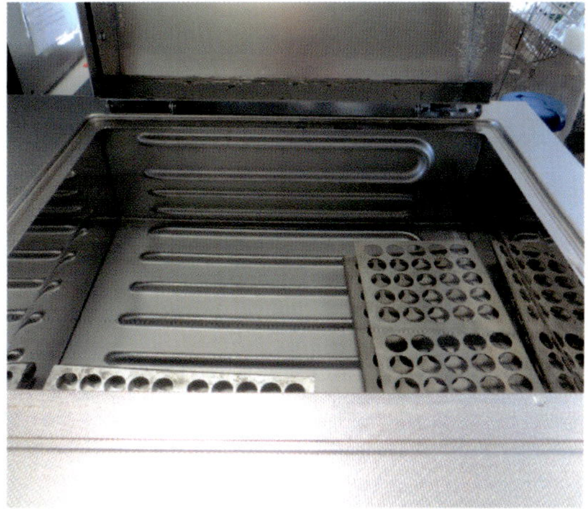

Figure 3. Inside of the water bath (37 °C).

Preparation of semen doses and semen storage

The semen should be gently added to the extender to prevent damage to the spermatozoa (Fig. 4).

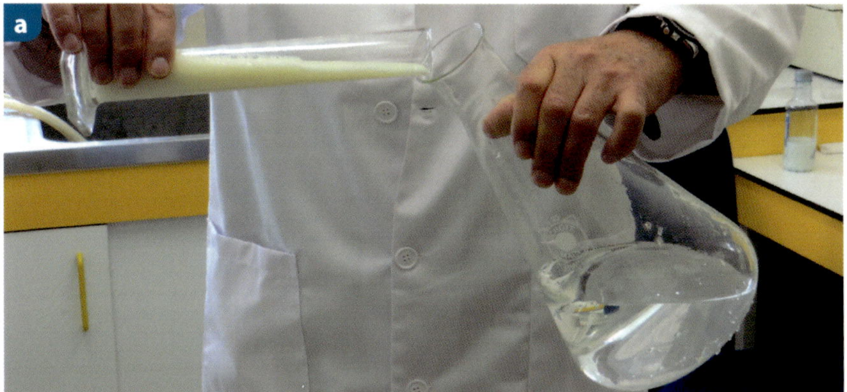

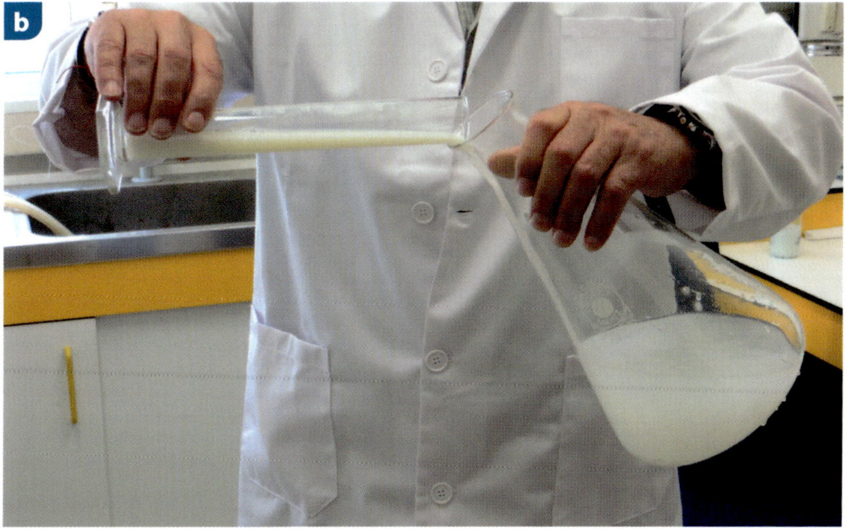

Figure 4. Semen and extender are gently mixed. Initial (a) and intermediate (b) steps.

The ideal dilution ratio is between 1:10 and 1:25 (Fig. 5). After this step, the diluted semen is transferred to bottles of 80–100 ml and part of the diluted semen is stored in sample tubes for control and evaluation of the entire process (Fig. 6).

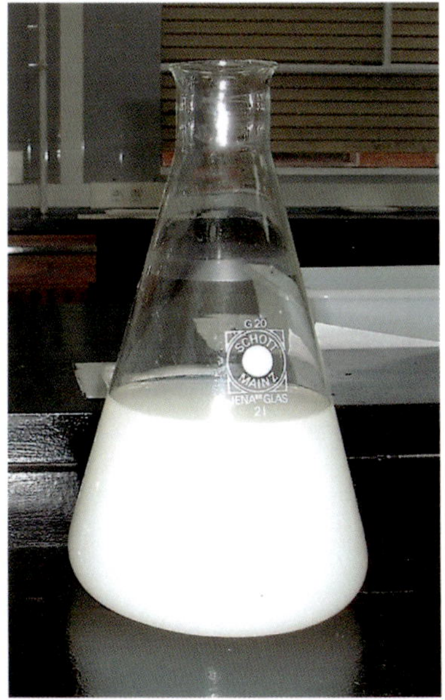

Figure 5. The optimum dilution ratio is between 1:10 and 1:25.

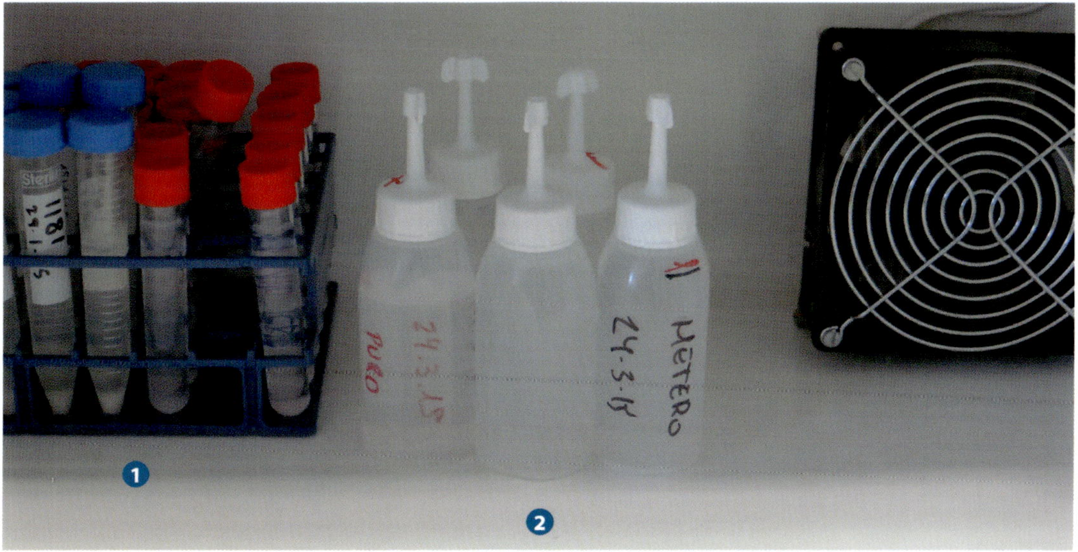

Figure 6. Control doses used to evaluate sperm parameters (1) and bottles of semen doses (80–100 ml) maintained at 15–17 °C (2).

Extension rate

To obtain a desired insemination dose (or bottle) of 3×10^9 spermatozoa/100 ml, the amount of extender required should be calculated as follows:

Total number of spermatozoa

Determined sperm concentration (see Chapter 5) $\times$ Ejaculate volume

↓

52×10^7 spermatozoa/ml $\times$ 125 ml = 65×10^9 total spermatozoa

Number of doses at required concentration

Total number of spermatozoa ÷ Desired extension rate

↓

65×10^9 spermatozoa ÷ 3×10^9 spermatozoa/dose = 16 doses

Total volume required

Number of doses × Volume of semen dose

16×100 ml = 1,600 ml total volume

Extender volume

Total volume – Ejaculate volume

1,600 ml – 125 ml = 1,475 ml of extender required

Therefore:

- Add 125 ml semen to 1,475 ml of extender.
- Transfer extended semen into 16 bottles (100 ml) to obtain 3×10^9 spermatozoa/dose.
- Finally, the temperature of the semen dose is gradually decreased from 20–25 °C to 15–17 °C over 90 to 150 minutes for subsequent refrigerated storage or transport (Fig. 7).

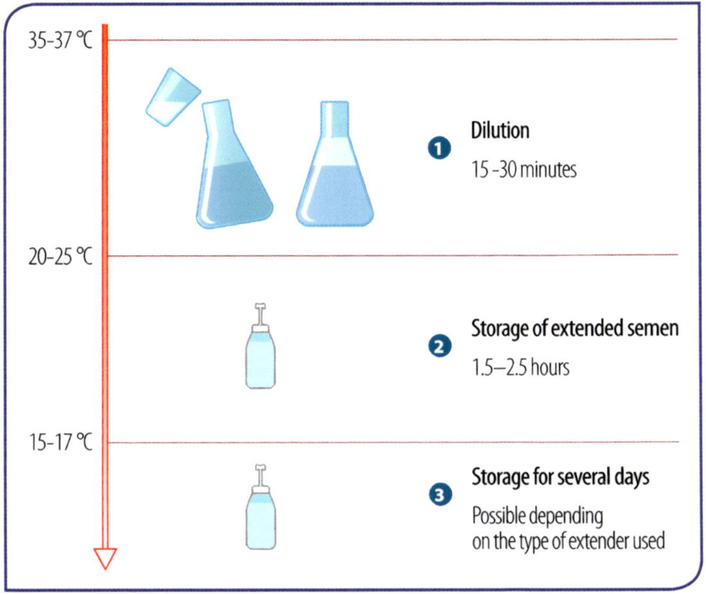

Figure 7. Appropriate temperatures for the collection, dilution, and storage of semen doses. It is very important to check sperm motility at each stage of the process. 1: dilution phase; 2: storage of extended semen (doses) phase; 3: storage phase (15-17 ºC).

Bottles stored in the refrigerator should be kept horizontal, as shown in Figure 8.

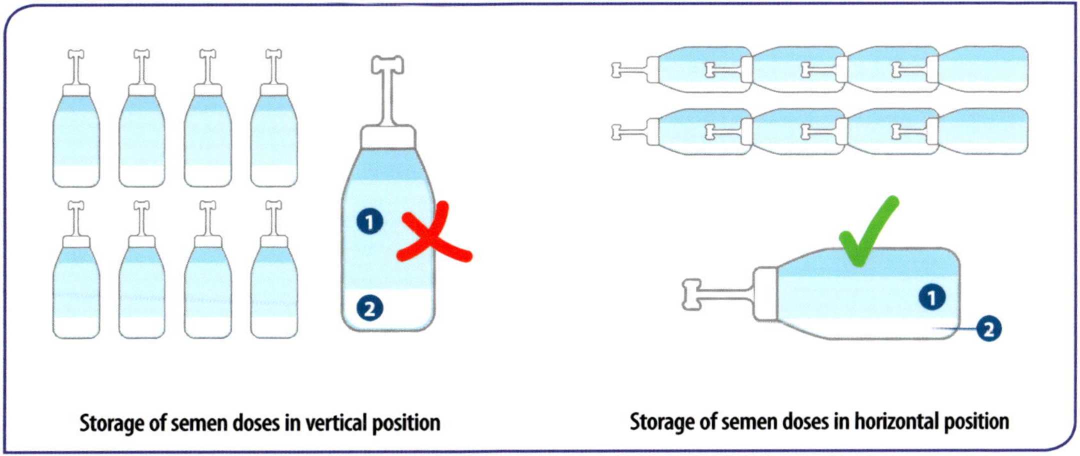

Figure 8. Position of bottles for storage at refrigerated temperatures (15–17 °C). 1: extender; 2: sperm sedimentation. Bottles should be maintained in horizontal position.

This guarantees a greater contact area between the spermatozoa and the extender, and prevents agglutination, ensuring better preservation and maintenance of the optimal fertilising capacity of the semen dose (Figs. 9 and 10). The bottles should be moved gently once or twice a day or every 12 hours.

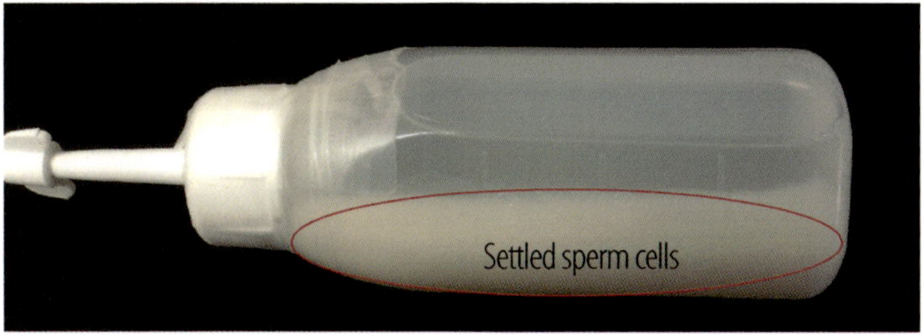

Figure 9. Storage in horizontal position allows for greater surface of contact between spermatozoa and extender.

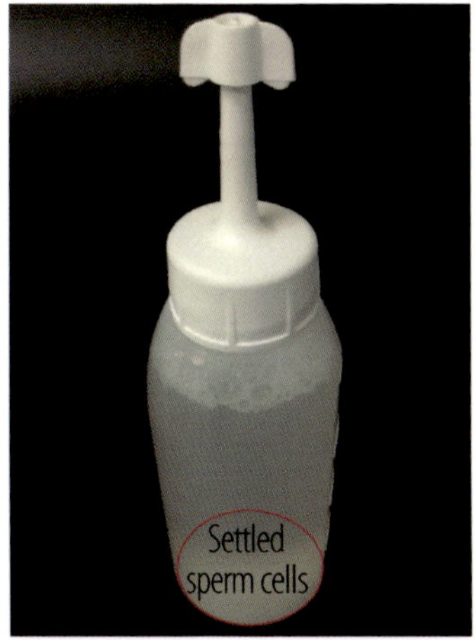

Figure 10. Storage in vertical position minimises contact surface between sperm cells and extender.

Figure 11 describes the different stages of boar semen dilution and storage.

In AICs that produce large numbers of semen doses this entire process, from dilution to bottling of the semen dose, is completely automated.

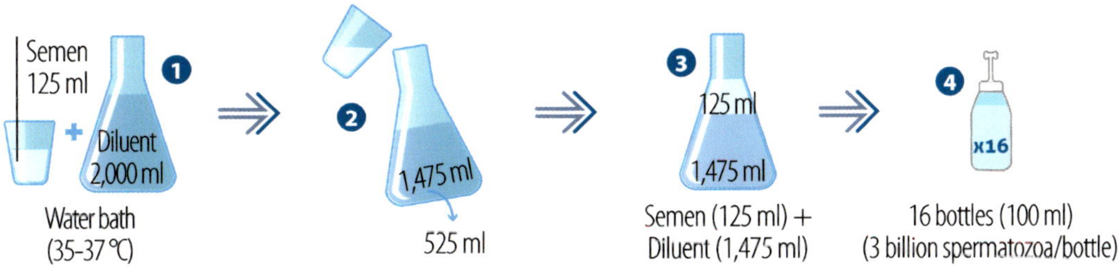

1. The temperature of the semen and extender should be the same (37 ºC).
2. Discard some diluent and add semen to the liquid extender.
3. The recommended semen:extender ratio is 1:10–1:25.
4. Storage of extended semen. The optimal storage temperature is 15–17 ºC.

Figure 11. Stages of boar semen dilution and storage.

References

Althouse GC. Optimizing productivity of the AI boar. https://projects.ncsu.edu/project/swine_extension/healthyhogs/book1997/althouse2.htm 1997. Consulted 8/October/16.

Cole HH, Cupps PT. Órganos reproductores masculinos y semen en *Reproducción de los animales domésticos*. Editoral Acribia. 1984; pp.192.

De Alba C, Grossfeld R. Pig Progress. www.PigProgress.net 2012; 28(7).

De Alba C. Optimización del uso de verracos de alto valor genético. http://www.infopork.com/2014/08/optimizaci-n-del-uso-de-verracos-de-alto-valor-gen-tico/. Consulted: 7/October/16.

Didion BA. Computer-assisted semen analysis and its utility for profiling boar semen samples. *Theriogenology* 2008, 70:1374–6.

Goldberg AM, Argenti LE, Faccin JE, Linck L, Santi M, Bernardi ML, Cardoso MR, Wentz I, Bortolozzo FP. Risk factors for bacterial contamination during boar semen collection. *Research in Veterinary Science.* 2013; 95 (2):362-367.

França LR, Avelar GF, Almeida FF. Spermatogenesis and sperm transit through the epididymis in mammals with emphasis on pigs. *Theriogenology* 2005, 63 300–318.

Hafez ESE. Anatomy of male reproduction in *Reproduction in farm animals.* 2000; 7th Edition (eds. B. Hafez and ESE Hafez), Lippincott Williams & Wilkins, Baltimore, Maryland, USA. doi: 10.1002/9781119265306.ch1

Hansen C, Vermeiden T, Vermeiden JPW, Simmet C, Day BC, Feitsma H. Comparison of FACSCount AF system, Improved Neubauer hemocytometer, Corning 254 photometer, Sperm Vision, Ulti Mate and Nucleo Counter SP-100 for determination of sperm concentration of boar semen. *Theriogenology.* 2006; 66:2188-2194.

Johnson LA, Weitze KF, Fiser P, Maxwell WMC. Storage of boar semen. *Animal Reproduction Science.* 2000; 62:143-172.

Knox, R. 2003. The anatomy and physiology of sperm production in boars. http://www.e-bookspdf.org/view/.

Knox, R. Semen processing, extending & storage for artificial insemination in swine. http://livestocktrail.illinois.edu/uploads/swinerepronet/papers/Semen%20Processing.pdf consultado: 20/October/16.

Kubus S.A. Manual de inseminación artificial porcina. 1999. Ed. KUBUS, S.A

Martín-Rillo S. Aportación al estudio de la congelación del semen de verraco. 1986. PhD thesis. University of Zaragoza. Spain.

Parrish JJ. Reproductive Physiology. http://www.ansci.wisc.edu/jjp1/ansci_repro/index.html. Consulted 19/December/16

PIC. Boar Stud Management Manual. 2015. http://na.picgenus.com/sites/genuspic_com/Uploads/Boar%20Manual.pdf consulted: 18/October/16.

Pursel VG, Johnson LA. Freezing of boar spermatozoa: Fertilizing capacity with concentrated semen and a new thawing procedure. *J Anim Sci.* 1975; 40:99-102.

Riesenbeck A. Review on international trade with boar semen. *Reprod Domest Anim.* 2011; 46:1–3.

Verstegen J, Iguer-Ouada M, Onclin K. Computer assisted semen analysers in andrology research and veterinary practice. *Theriogenology*. 2001; 57:149-179.